From Chaos to Calm

Mindful Parenting Practices for Busy Moms

by Nova Reign

About Me

Hi, I'm Katie—a mom of three boys and a bonus son, juggling the beautiful chaos of motherhood with a full-time work-from-home job. My boys are 12, 4, 2, and a newborn, so yes, I'm 100% a boy mom living in a house that's rarely quiet (or clean, let's be honest). Life here is a mix of toy dinosaurs and cars, kids running around screaming, stickiness, and lots of snacks—oh, and did I mention I have ADHD? I'm also about 99% sure my 4-year-old does too, which keeps things... interesting! Parenting in our home feels like a marathon some days and a whirlwind others, but in the middle of all this momma madness, I've started embracing mindfulness. I put together this book because, like you, I'm learning to slow down, stay present, and find calm in the chaos—not just for my kids, but for myself. If you're a busy mom trying to keep it all together while creating meaningful moments, you're not alone. We're all figuring this out as we go. Let's take it one mindful step at a time!

Table Of Contents

Introduction: Why Mindful Parenting Matters

Parenting is one of the most fulfilling yet overwhelming journeys in life. From sleepless nights to busy days juggling work and family, the chaos of daily responsibilities often leaves moms feeling stretched thin and disconnected from their own sense of self. Many mothers find themselves caught in a constant cycle of doing, rarely pausing to simply be. It's in these moments of overwhelm that the need for mindfulness becomes clear.

From Chaos to Calm is not just another parenting guide—it's a lifeline for moms who want to reclaim their peace and joy who are constantly on the go. This book isn't about being the perfect mom or creating a picture-perfect home. Instead, it's about embracing imperfection, showing up with intention, and building meaningful connections with your children, your family, and, most importantly, yourself. The journey to mindful parenting begins with small, intentional steps that ripple outward, transforming your family life one moment at a time.

In the pages ahead, you'll discover simple yet impactful strategies to help you navigate the challenges of parenting with greater clarity and calm. From practical tips to mindful routines, this book will show you how to create space for connection, manage stressful moments, and nurture your own well-being. Whether you're looking to strengthen your bond with your children or simply find a way to breathe amidst the chaos, this book is your guide. Together, we'll uncover the path to a more intentional, harmonious way of living—one step at a time.

Chapter 1: The Foundations of Mindfulness

What is Mindfulness?

Mindfulness is the practice of being fully present in the moment—acknowledging your thoughts, feelings, and experiences without judgment. For busy moms, this means carving out moments to connect deeply with yourself, your children, and your surroundings. In a world filled with distractions, mindfulness offers a beacon of calm, helping you navigate the challenges of parenting with patience and understanding.

At its core, mindfulness encourages us to slow down and pay attention to the small details that often go overlooked— like the way your child's laughter rings out during playtime or the warmth of their hand in yours during a quiet moment. These moments, often overlooked in the rush of daily life, become cherished memories when we practice mindfulness.

Incorporating mindfulness into your parenting doesn't require significant time or resources. Simple practices like deep breathing, mindful listening, or even savoring a cup of tea can provide moments of peace and recharge your spirit, helping you face motherhood's demands with greater ease. Remember, mindfulness isn't about perfection—it's about progress and finding joy in the present. Every small step leads to a more balanced, fulfilling parenting experience.

The Benefits of Mindfulness for Parents

Mindfulness offers transformative benefits, especially for busy moms. Engaging in mindful practices can reduce stress and anxiety, creating a more peaceful home. By taking moments each day to connect with the present, you cultivate a sense of calm that influences your interactions with your children. Mindfulness helps you approach challenges with clarity, fostering resilience and patience.

One of the most significant benefits of mindfulness is enhanced emotional regulation. By practicing mindfulness, you learn to observe your thoughts and feelings without judgment or reaction. This skill is invaluable during parenting, where emotions can run high. Pausing to breathe and reflect allows you to respond with empathy rather than frustration, strengthening the parent-child bond.

Mindfulness also deepens your connection with your children. In today's fast-paced world, distractions can lead to missed opportunities for meaningful interactions. When you incorporate mindfulness into your routine, you're able to fully engage with your children—whether during playtime, mealtime, or simple moments of connection. This presence helps children feel valued and secure.

Additionally, mindfulness supports self-care. As a busy mom, you might prioritize your children's needs above your own, leading to burnout. By dedicating time to mindfulness practices like meditation or mindful walking, you replenish your emotional and physical reserves. This self-nurturing practice not only benefits you but also models the importance of self-care for your children.

Finally, mindfulness encourages a positive mindset. Parenting can be challenging, but mindfulness fosters gratitude, helping you shift from focusing on what's wrong to appreciating what's going right. This positive perspective creates a culture of optimism and resilience in your family.

Mindfulness vs. Multitasking

In today's fast-paced world, parents often feel the pressure to do it all at once. Juggling work, family responsibilities, and personal time, many mothers find themselves caught in the whirlwind of multitasking. While it may seem efficient to handle several tasks simultaneously, research shows that multitasking can actually lead to increased stress and decreased productivity. By embracing mindfulness, parents can shift their focus from doing many things at once to fully engaging in one task at a time, allowing for a more peaceful and fulfilling parenting experience.

Mindfulness is the practice of being present and fully engaged in the moment, without judgment. When parents adopt mindfulness, they cultivate a greater awareness of their thoughts, emotions, and surroundings. This practice can transform daily routines into meaningful interactions with children. For instance, instead of trying to cook dinner while helping with homework and checking emails, mindfulness encourages parents to focus on one activity at a time. This not only enhances the quality of the work being done but also allows for deeper connections with children, fostering a sense of calm in the home.

The drawbacks of multitasking are particularly evident in parenting. When we divide our attention, we often miss out on precious moments with our children. The laughter during playtime, the curiosity during homework, and the simple joy of sharing a meal can all be overshadowed by the constant urge to multitask. By recognizing these moments and choosing to be present, parents can create lasting memories and strengthen their relationships with their children. Mindfulness helps to slow down the chaotic pace of life, encouraging parents to appreciate the beauty in everyday interactions.

Transitioning from a multitasking mindset to a more mindful approach takes practice and patience. Parents can start small by dedicating specific time to focus solely on their children. Setting aside technology-free moments, such as during meals or bedtime stories, can significantly enhance the quality of these experiences. As parents become more attuned to the benefits of being present, they may find that their overall stress levels decrease, and their ability to connect with their children improves. This shift not only fosters a sense of peace but also models healthy habits for children, teaching them the value of mindfulness in their own lives.

Overall, the journey from chaos to calm parenting begins with the choice to prioritize mindfulness over multitasking. By committing to being present in each moment, parents can create a nurturing environment that promotes emotional well-being for both themselves and their children. As busy moms embrace this mindful approach, they will discover that less truly can be more—more joy, more connection, and more peace. It's a powerful reminder that in the world of parenting, the moments we choose to focus on can have the most profound impact.

Chapter 2: Embracing the Journey

Understanding the Role of Mindfulness in Parenting

Parenting presents countless moments of chaos, from toddler tantrums to teenage mood swings. Mindfulness helps parents approach these situations with calm and clarity, creating a nurturing environment where both parents and children can thrive

When emotions run high—whether during a toddler's meltdown or a teenager's rebellious outburst—mindfulness teaches parents to pause and respond with empathy instead of reacting impulsively. For example, before addressing a tantrum, take three deep breaths and reflect on your child's perspective. This intentional pause not only helps regulate your own emotions but also models healthy emotional habits for your children.

Mindfulness also invites parents to be fully present during family moments. Instead of letting distractions pull you away, focus wholeheartedly on activities with your children, like reading together or playing a game. For example, during meals, put aside devices and engage in a conversation about your child's day. These moments of presence foster deeper connections, making children feel valued and loved.

Finally, mindfulness empowers parents to embrace self-compassion. Parenting comes with inevitable challenges, and mistakes are part of the journey. By acknowledging your imperfections with kindness, you can let go of guilt and approach parenting with a lighter heart. For instance, when you have a hard day, remind yourself, "I'm doing my best, and that's enough." Mindfulness in parenting is about progress, not perfection. Each small effort to practice presence, empathy, and self-compassion brings you closer to a more harmonious and fulfilling family life.

The Importance of Self-Care for Busy Moms

In the whirlwind of motherhood, it's easy to overlook your own needs amid the chaos of daily responsibilities. Yet, self-care is not a luxury; it's a necessity that lays the foundation for a healthier, more balanced life. When you prioritize your well-being, you cultivate the energy and resilience needed to care for your family. Remember, you cannot pour from an empty cup—nurturing yourself is essential for nurturing your children.

Regular self-care reduces stress and promotes emotional well-being, providing an opportunity to recharge, reflect, and reconnect with your identity outside of being a mom. Whether it's savoring a quiet moment with a book, enjoying a warm bath, or practicing mindfulness, these small acts of self-kindness can significantly improve your mood and mindset. By dedicating time to yourself, you create a ripple effect that enhances your interactions with your children and fosters a more positive home environment.

Self-care also empowers you and reinforces your sense of self-worth. When you set aside time for activities that bring you joy, you send a powerful message to both yourself and your children: *your needs are important and deserve attention.* Modeling this kind of self-respect teaches your children invaluable lessons about valuing their own mental health and well-being. By prioritizing self-care, you inspire them to develop habits of mindfulness and self-compassion that will benefit them for a lifetime.

Incorporating self-care doesn't have to be daunting. Small, manageable practices can make a significant difference. Consider dedicating just ten minutes a day to something that replenishes your spirit—whether it's breathing exercises, a short walk, or simply savoring a cup of tea in peace. These brief but meaningful moments remind you of your worth and help you maintain calm amidst life's chaos.

Ultimately, embracing self-care is a crucial step toward achieving the balance every busy mom seeks. It enables you to show up fully for your family while also honoring your own needs. By recognizing the importance of self-care, you empower yourself to create a harmonious environment where both you and your children can thrive. Taking care of yourself isn't just a gift to you; it's a gift to your entire family, fostering a dynamic of love, support, and understanding that will last for generations.

Setting Intentions for a Calmer Life

Setting intentions is a powerful practice that can transform the chaos of daily life into a more peaceful and purposeful existence. As busy parents, especially mothers, it's easy to get swept away by the demands of everyday responsibilities. By consciously setting intentions for a calmer life, you create a roadmap that guides your thoughts and actions, helping you navigate through challenges with clarity and tranquility. This practice encourages you to pause, reflect, and choose how you want to show up for yourself and your family.

To begin the process of setting intentions, it's helpful to create a dedicated space for reflection. This could be a quiet corner in your home, a cozy nook with a favorite chair, or even a place in nature where you feel grounded. Take a few moments each day to sit in this space, close your eyes, and breathe deeply. Allow your mind to settle, letting go of distractions. As you breathe, think about what a calmer life looks like for you. What feelings do you want to cultivate? What actions can you take to align with that vision? Writing down your thoughts can provide clarity and serve as a reminder in moments of stress.

Once you have a clearer picture of your intentions, it's important to articulate them in a positive manner. Instead of focusing on what you want to eliminate, frame your intentions around what you want to invite into your life. For instance, rather than saying, "I don't want to feel overwhelmed," you might express, "I intend to embrace moments of peace and joy." This shift in language not only makes your intentions more empowering but also helps to reinforce a mindset that seeks out positivity amidst the chaos.

As you progress in this practice, remember that setting intentions is not a one-time event but a continual journey. Life will inevitably bring challenges, and it's during these times that your intentions can be most beneficial. When you feel the weight of stress, revisit your intentions and allow them to serve as an anchor. Reflect on how you can embody these intentions in your daily routines, whether it's through mindful breathing, taking breaks, or simply reminding yourself to choose calm in the face of turbulence.

Finally, share your intentions with others, whether it's your partner, children, or friends. Discussing your goals can create a supportive environment where everyone is encouraged to pursue their own peaceful practices. By modeling intentional living, you inspire those around you to embrace mindfulness and contribute to a collective sense of calm. As you journey through the beautiful chaos of parenting, remember that setting intentions for a calmer life is a gift you give not only to yourself but also to your family, fostering a nurturing and serene atmosphere for everyone.

Chapter 3: Creating a Mindful Home Environment

Decluttering for Peace of Mind

Decluttering for peace of mind starts with understanding that our physical environment profoundly affects our mental state. As parents, our homes can often become overwhelmed with toys, clothes, and various items that seem to multiply overnight. The chaos can lead to stress and anxiety, making it harder to focus on the meaningful moments we want to share with our children. By taking small, intentional steps to declutter our surroundings, we can create a serene atmosphere that promotes mindfulness and relaxation.

Begin by setting aside just a few minutes each day to tackle one small area. This could be a single drawer, a shelf, or even a corner of a room. The key is to start small, which helps prevent feelings of overwhelm. As you sort through items, ask yourself if each piece serves a purpose or brings you joy. If not, consider donating or discarding it. This process not only lightens your physical load but also clears your mind, allowing you to focus more on the present moment with your children.

Involve your kids in the decluttering process whenever possible. This not only teaches them valuable lessons about organization and responsibility but also helps them understand the importance of creating a peaceful environment. Make it a fun activity by turning it into a game or setting a timer for a quick decluttering challenge. As they see their contributions making a difference, they will feel empowered and more likely to keep their spaces tidy in the future.

Once you've established a decluttering routine, maintain it by regularly reassessing your belongings. Life changes, and so do our needs and preferences. Develop a habit of evaluating items every few months, ensuring that your space remains a reflection of your current lifestyle. This ongoing practice will prevent clutter from building up again and will keep your home feeling light and open, fostering a sense of calm for you and your family.

As you create a more organized space, take a moment to appreciate the peace it brings. A decluttered home often leads to a decluttered mind, allowing you to engage more fully in the precious moments of parenting. Celebrate your progress, no matter how small, and recognize that each step towards a more organized environment is a step towards a more mindful and joyful parenting experience. Embrace the journey, and remember that by prioritizing your peace of mind, you are also nurturing a harmonious space for your children to thrive.

Designing Spaces for Calm and Connection

Creating spaces that foster calm and connection is essential for parents looking to cultivate mindfulness in their homes. The environment we inhabit significantly influences our emotional state and interactions with our children. By intentionally designing spaces that promote tranquility, we can create a nurturing atmosphere that encourages open communication and deeper connections. Simple changes can transform our homes into sanctuaries where both parents and children feel safe, relaxed, and connected.

Start by decluttering your living areas. Clutter can be overwhelming and distracting, creating a chaotic environment that interferes with mindfulness. Take a moment to assess your spaces and remove items that no longer serve a purpose or bring joy. Involve your children in this process; it not only teaches them valuable organizational skills but also reinforces the idea that our surroundings can reflect our emotional well-being. As you streamline your environment, you may notice a newfound sense of calm washing over your home.

Incorporate elements that engage the senses and promote relaxation. Soft lighting, soothing colors, and natural materials can create a warm atmosphere that invites connection. Consider adding comfortable seating areas where you can spend quality time with your children, fostering conversations and shared experiences. Introduce plants or nature-inspired decor to bring a sense of tranquility indoors. These small touches not only enhance the aesthetic appeal but also create a peaceful backdrop for mindful parenting practices.

Establish designated areas for mindfulness activities, such as reading, meditation, or creative play. Having specific spaces dedicated to these practices encourages everyone in the family to engage in them regularly. Create a cozy reading nook filled with books that inspire imagination and curiosity. Set up a quiet corner with cushions and calming visuals for meditation or reflection. By carving out these intentional spaces, you signal to your family that nurturing their emotional health is a priority, fostering a culture of mindfulness in your home.

Finally, remember the importance of connection in these spaces. Arrange seating to encourage face-to-face interactions, and make time for family rituals that promote bonding, such as shared meals or game nights. Use these moments to practice active listening and open communication, allowing everyone to express their thoughts and feelings. As you cultivate an environment designed for calm and connection, you empower your family to embrace mindfulness together, reinforcing the lessons of love, support, and understanding that will last a lifetime.

Incorporating Nature into Your Home

Incorporating nature into your home can transform your living space into a serene sanctuary that nurtures both you and your children. As busy parents, it can be challenging to find moments of peace amidst the chaos of daily life. By inviting elements of the natural world indoors, you create a calming environment that fosters mindfulness and connection. Simple changes, such as adding houseplants, can purify the air and enhance your mood, making your home a more inviting space for relaxation and connection.

Consider starting with plants that are easy to care for and suitable for indoor environments. Species like snake plants, pothos, and peace lilies not only thrive with minimal attention but also contribute to a healthier home atmosphere. Involving your children in the process of selecting and caring for these plants can be a wonderful bonding experience. Teach them about the importance of nature and how plants can improve our well-being. This shared responsibility can instill a sense of accomplishment and teach valuable lessons about nurturing living things.

Creating nature-inspired decor is another effective way to bring the outside in. Use natural materials like wood, stone, and textiles that mimic the colors and textures of the outdoors. Displaying artwork featuring landscapes or natural scenes can evoke a sense of tranquility and remind everyone of the beauty found in nature. You might also consider incorporating natural light into your home design by keeping windows unobstructed and using sheer curtains. This simple adjustment can brighten your space and enhance your family's mood.

In addition to plants and decor, you can integrate nature by introducing sensory experiences that evoke the outdoors. Consider using essential oils or candles with earthy scents like pine or lavender to create a calming atmosphere. Natural sounds, such as recordings of birds chirping or gentle water flowing, can also promote relaxation during family activities. These sensory elements not only enrich your environment but also help cultivate mindfulness, encouraging everyone to pause and appreciate the present moment together.

Finally, remember that your home is a reflection of your family's values and lifestyle. By intentionally incorporating nature into your space, you are modeling mindful living for your children. Encourage them to explore the outdoors, even in small ways, like taking nature walks or creating a garden. These experiences can deepen their connection to the world around them and foster a sense of peace and calm that will benefit the entire family. Embrace this journey of integrating nature into your home, and watch as it transforms your parenting experience into one filled with joy, connection, and tranquility.

Chapter 4: Mindful Morning Routines

Waking Up with Intention

Waking up with intention sets the tone for your entire day, especially as a busy parent. In the early moments of the morning, before the demands of the day unfold, you have the opportunity to cultivate a mindset that can carry you through the chaos. Instead of diving straight into your to-do list, take a few moments to pause and breathe. This simple act of mindfulness can create a ripple effect, allowing you to respond to daily challenges with greater calmness and clarity.

Begin your day with a short ritual that resonates with you. It could be as simple as enjoying a cup of tea in silence, journaling your thoughts, or practicing a few stretches. This intentional start not only grounds you but also reminds you of your values and goals. When you infuse your morning with purpose, you set a foundation for patience and presence, allowing you to navigate your parenting journey with a centered heart and mind.

Consider incorporating affirmations into your morning routine. Positive affirmations can serve as powerful reminders of your strength and capabilities as a parent. By affirming your intentions for the day—like patience, love, or resilience—you create a mental framework that encourages you to embody these qualities throughout your interactions with your children. This practice reinforces the idea that you are not just reacting to the chaos but actively shaping your experience with mindful choices.

As you embrace the practice of waking up with intention, remember that it's okay to start small. You don't need to overhaul your entire morning routine at once. Perhaps begin with just five minutes dedicated to mindfulness. Gradually, as you become more comfortable, you can expand this time or introduce additional practices that resonate with you. Celebrate these small victories, as they contribute to a larger transformation in how you experience each day.

Finally, recognize that waking up with intention is a journey, not a destination. Some days will feel easier than others, and that's perfectly okay. Offer yourself grace during those hectic mornings when chaos seems to reign. The key is to return to your practice whenever you can, allowing it to evolve alongside your needs as a parent. Each new day presents a fresh start, a chance to infuse your parenting with mindfulness and intention, ultimately leading you closer to the calm you seek amidst the busyness of life.

Mindful Breakfast Practices

Mindful breakfast practices can set a positive tone for the entire day, creating a peaceful and nurturing environment for both parents and children. As busy moms, mornings can often feel chaotic, filled with rushing and stress. By incorporating mindfulness into your breakfast routine, you can transform this daily ritual into a moment of connection and calm. Start by dedicating a few moments each morning to breathe deeply and ground yourself. This simple act can help you approach the day with a clearer mind and a more open heart.

Prepare your breakfast mindfully by engaging all your senses in the process. As you chop, stir, or toast, take note of the colors, textures, and aromas of the ingredients. Allow yourself to truly experience the act of cooking, making it a sensory adventure rather than a chore. Involve your children in this practice by encouraging them to describe what they see and smell. This not only fosters a sense of teamwork but also helps them develop a deeper appreciation for food and the effort that goes into preparing it.

Consider creating a breakfast ritual that everyone in the family can look forward to. Whether it's a special dish on certain days or a fun way to serve the food, rituals can add an element of joy and anticipation to the morning routine. You might choose to set the table together, lighting a candle or playing soft music as you enjoy your meal. These small gestures can elevate breakfast from a rushed obligation to a cherished family moment, allowing everyone to feel more connected and present.

As you sit down to eat, practice gratitude by taking a moment to reflect on the nourishment before you. Encourage your children to share what they are thankful for, fostering a sense of appreciation and mindfulness around food. This practice not only enhances the experience of breakfast but also instills valuable lessons about gratitude and mindfulness in your children. A simple "thank you" can create a ripple effect of positivity that carries throughout the day.

Finally, remember that mindful breakfast practices are not just about the food but also about the conversations that happen around the table. Use this time to connect with your children, asking open-ended questions about their dreams, fears, or plans for the day. Listening attentively and engaging in meaningful dialogue can deepen your bond and create a safe space for your children to express themselves. By prioritizing these mindful moments, you are nurturing not only their well-being but your own, transforming breakfast into a powerful practice of calm and connection.

Setting the Tone for the Day

Setting the tone for the day begins the moment you wake up. As a busy mom, it's easy to feel overwhelmed by the demands of the day ahead, but taking a few moments each morning to cultivate a positive mindset can transform your experience. Start by creating a morning ritual that resonates with you, whether it's a few minutes of deep breathing, sipping your favorite tea, or journaling your intentions. These small acts of self-care not only ground you but also set a peaceful foundation for your family.

As the day progresses, mindfulness can help you stay centered amidst the chaos. Consider incorporating simple practices, such as pausing to take a deep breath whenever you feel tension rising. This can be especially useful during hectic mornings when everyone is trying to get out the door. By modeling these moments of calm, you not only benefit yourself but also teach your children the importance of managing their emotions and finding stillness in the midst of busyness.

Creating a positive atmosphere at home goes beyond individual practices. Involve your children in setting the tone for the day by encouraging them to share their feelings and aspirations each morning. This open dialogue fosters a sense of connection and helps everyone feel heard. You might establish a family tradition, like sharing one positive affirmation or gratitude before breakfast. This simple act can uplift spirits and reinforce a culture of positivity in your home.

Another powerful way to set the tone is through the environment you create. Consider how your surroundings impact your mood. A tidy space filled with natural light, inviting colors, and elements that inspire joy can make a significant difference. Involve your children in this process by allowing them to contribute their ideas about decor or organization. When everyone has a stake in the environment, it cultivates a sense of ownership and pride that can enhance the overall atmosphere of your home.

Finally, remember that setting the tone is an ongoing practice. Each day presents new opportunities to foster a calm and loving environment. Embrace the fluctuations that come with parenting, knowing that it's normal to have challenging days. By consistently returning to your mindful practices, you'll cultivate resilience within yourself and your family. Celebrate the small victories and remain open to change, allowing each day to be a new chance to create a harmonious start for you and your children.

Chapter 5: Mindful Communication with Children

Active Listening Techniques

Active listening is a powerful tool in mindful parenting that can transform the way you connect with your children. It goes beyond simply hearing their words; it involves fully engaging with their thoughts and feelings. As a parent, when you practice active listening, you create a safe space for your child to express themselves. This practice not only strengthens your bond but also fosters trust, allowing your child to feel valued and understood.

One effective technique for active listening is to maintain eye contact. When you look your child in the eye, you communicate that they have your undivided attention. This simple act can significantly enhance their willingness to share their feelings and thoughts. Additionally, try to minimize distractions during conversations. Set aside your phone, turn off the television, and focus solely on what your child is saying. This mindful approach shows them that their words are important and deserving of your full presence.

Reflective listening is another valuable technique that can deepen your connection. After your child shares their thoughts, paraphrase what they've said to confirm your understanding. For example, you might say, "It sounds like you're feeling frustrated about your homework." This not only clarifies their feelings but also encourages them to elaborate further. By reflecting on their emotions and thoughts, you help them feel heard and validated, which is crucial for their emotional development.

Encouraging open-ended questions can also enhance active listening. Instead of asking questions that lead to simple yes or no answers, invite your child to share more by asking questions like, "How did that make you feel?" or "What do you think will happen next?" These types of questions stimulate deeper conversations, allowing your child to explore their emotions and thoughts more freely. The more you encourage this type of dialogue, the more comfortable they will become in expressing themselves.

Finally, practice patience during conversations. Sometimes, children need time to articulate their thoughts or may struggle with expressing their feelings. Give them the space to gather their thoughts without interrupting. Your patience will demonstrate that you are truly interested in understanding them, which can encourage them to open up even more. By implementing these active listening techniques, you will not only enhance your relationship with your child but also nurture their emotional intelligence, paving the way for a more peaceful and connected family dynamic.

Practicing Empathy in Daily Interactions

Practicing empathy in daily interactions is a transformative approach for parents striving to create a nurturing and supportive environment for their children. Empathy allows you to connect deeply with your child, helping them feel seen, understood, and valued. When you practice empathy, you move beyond simply reacting to behavior and start tuning into the emotions and experiences driving it. This shift in perspective leads to more meaningful conversations, stronger bonds, and a more fulfilling parenting journey.

Incorporating empathy into everyday routines doesn't have to be complicated. For example, when your child is frustrated with a task, resist the urge to immediately solve the problem for them. Instead, pause and ask how they're feeling about the challenge. Encourage them to articulate their thoughts and emotions. This approach not only helps them navigate difficulties but also reinforces the idea that vulnerability is okay. By creating a safe space for emotional expression, you empower your child to develop emotional intelligence, a skill that will benefit them throughout their life.

Another way to practice empathy is through action, such as involving your child in decisions that affect them. For example, if your child resists getting ready for bed, instead of enforcing the routine with frustration, invite their input: *"I know bedtime can feel rushed. What would make it feel better for you? Maybe we can choose a story together or decide on a special bedtime song."* Including your child in decisions not only shows respect for their feelings but also fosters collaboration and mutual understanding.

You can also model empathy by acknowledging their physical needs with care and attentiveness. For instance, if your child is whining because they're overtired, instead of saying, *"Stop whining,"* try responding with compassion: *"You seem really tired right now. Let's get you comfortable and rest a little."* This teaches them to recognize and respond to their own needs with kindness, reinforcing that their emotions and physical states are valid and important.

Another powerful way to model empathy is by sharing your own feelings and experiences. When appropriate, let your child in on your emotions, especially when they parallel challenges they might face. For instance, if you've had a tough day at work, you might say, *"I felt really frustrated today because something didn't go as planned, but talking about it is helping me feel better."* This kind of transparency strengthens your relationship by showing your child that even adults face struggles. It also demonstrates that empathy is a two-way street, where understanding flows both ways.

Finally, remember that empathy is a lifelong practice. Each interaction with your child is an opportunity to deepen your connection and support their emotional well-being. Celebrate the small victories—whether it's a heartfelt conversation or a moment of mutual understanding. As you consistently practice empathy, you create a calm, loving atmosphere where your child can thrive, ultimately fostering a more peaceful and connected family life.

Encouraging Open Dialogue

Encouraging open dialogue within the family is essential for fostering a nurturing environment where each member feels valued and heard. As busy parents, it can be easy to overlook the importance of communication, yet creating a space for open conversations can significantly enhance your family's emotional well-being. When children know they can express their thoughts and feelings without judgment, they develop confidence and a sense of security. This not only strengthens relationships but also encourages emotional intelligence as they learn to articulate their feelings and understand those of others.

One effective way to promote open dialogue is to establish regular family meetings. These gatherings can be informal and flexible, allowing everyone to share updates about their week, discuss challenges, and celebrate achievements. By setting aside dedicated time for conversation, you signal to your children that their voices matter. Additionally, these meetings can be an opportunity to practice active listening, where you model how to engage with others' perspectives thoughtfully. Encourage your children to share their thoughts openly, reinforcing that every opinion is valid and worthy of consideration.

Creating a safe space for dialogue also involves being present and attentive during conversations. When your child approaches you with a concern or a question, try to put aside distractions and give them your full attention. This small gesture can make a significant difference in how they perceive their ability to communicate with you. Acknowledge their feelings, validate their experiences, and respond with empathy. This practice not only strengthens your bond but also teaches your children the importance of being present with others and cultivating mindfulness in their interactions.

Encouragement is key when fostering open dialogue. Praise your children for expressing themselves, even when their opinions differ from yours. This validation helps them understand that varying viewpoints can coexist peacefully within a family. Use reflective listening techniques by paraphrasing what they've said, which shows that you are actively engaged in the conversation. This approach not only reinforces their willingness to share but also encourages critical thinking as they learn to articulate their thoughts more clearly.

Lastly, remember that open dialogue is a continuous process that requires patience and practice. It may take time for your children to fully embrace this culture of communication, especially if they are accustomed to a more reserved environment. Be persistent in your efforts to encourage discussions, and remain open to feedback about how they feel during these conversations. By nurturing this open dialogue, you create a calm and supportive atmosphere that promotes emotional growth and strengthens family connections, making your parenting journey more fulfilling and enriching.

Chapter 6: Mindful Playtime

The Importance of Play in Child Development

Play is a vital component of child development, serving as a natural way for children to learn about themselves and the world around them. Through play, children engage their imagination, creativity, and problem-solving skills. It allows them to explore their limits, understand social interactions, and develop emotional resilience. As parents, recognizing the significance of play can empower us to create environments that foster these essential skills, ultimately leading to well-rounded and confident children.

When children play, they naturally experiment with different roles and scenarios, which helps them understand complex concepts such as empathy and cooperation. Role-playing games, for instance, enable them to step into someone else's shoes, promoting social awareness and emotional intelligence. By encouraging our children to engage in various forms of play, we can help them develop important interpersonal skills that will serve them throughout their lives. This is a beautiful opportunity to nurture their ability to connect with others and build meaningful relationships.

Moreover, play is not just beneficial for cognitive and social development but also for physical health. Active play, such as running, jumping, or climbing, helps children develop their motor skills and coordination. It also instills a sense of adventure and confidence in their physical abilities. As busy moms, we can incorporate mindful practices into playtime by encouraging outdoor activities, which not only promote physical health but also allow our children to experience the calming effects of nature. This connection to the outdoors can be a source of joy and relaxation for both parents and children.

Mindful play also provides a unique opportunity for bonding between parents and children. When we actively participate in our child's play, we create cherished memories and deepen our connection. This shared experience fosters trust and communication, allowing our children to feel safe and supported in expressing their thoughts and feelings. By setting aside time for playful interaction, we not only contribute to their development but also enhance our relationship, making parenting a more joyful and harmonious journey.

Incorporating play into our daily routines does not have to be a complicated task. Simple, everyday moments can be transformed into playful interactions that promote learning and connection. Whether it's through imaginative storytelling, building forts, or playing games, these moments can significantly impact our children's emotional and cognitive well-being. As we embrace the importance of play, we create a nurturing atmosphere that encourages growth, creativity, and happiness, ultimately leading to a more peaceful and fulfilling parenting experience.

Engaging Fully in Play

Engaging fully in play is a transformative experience for both parents and children. It allows for genuine connections to be forged as you immerse yourself in the world of your child. When you set aside distractions, such as phones and household tasks, and actively participate in play, you create an environment where your child feels valued and understood. This commitment to being present can enhance your relationship, making it easier to navigate the challenges of parenting while cultivating a sense of joy and fulfillment.

To engage fully in play, it's essential to adopt a mindset of curiosity and openness. This means letting go of preconceived notions about how play should look or what activities are deemed appropriate. Instead, embrace your child's imagination and follow their lead. Whether it's building block towers, playing dress-up, or exploring outdoors, allowing yourself to be swept away in their enthusiasm can lead to moments of pure delight. This approach not only strengthens your bond but also fosters your child's creativity and confidence.

Mindfulness plays a crucial role in the process of engaging fully in play. By grounding yourself in the present moment, you can appreciate the small joys that come from simply being with your child. Take a deep breath, observe their laughter, and savor the sounds and sights around you. This mindful presence allows you to respond to your child's needs more effectively, creating a supportive atmosphere where they feel safe to express themselves. Remember, your engagement can significantly influence their emotional well-being and development.

Incorporating play into your daily routine can also serve as a powerful tool for stress relief. When you engage in play, you're not just spending time with your child; you're giving yourself permission to let go of adult worries and responsibilities, even if just for a moment. This can be a refreshing break from the chaos of daily life, allowing you to recharge your spirit and approach parenting with renewed energy. Embrace these playful moments as opportunities to nurture both your child and yourself.

Ultimately, engaging fully in play is a gift that enriches family life. It teaches children the importance of connection, creativity, and joy while providing parents with a deeper understanding of their child's world. By prioritizing playtime, you cultivate an atmosphere of love and laughter that can make the chaos of parenting feel more manageable. So, take a deep breath, dive into the fun, and allow yourself to be a joyful participant in your child's adventures.

Creative Activities for Mindfulness

Creative activities can serve as powerful tools for cultivating mindfulness in both parents and children. Engaging in these activities not only promotes relaxation but also fosters a deeper connection between you and your child. As you embark on this journey together, remember that the goal is not perfection but presence. Embrace the moments you share, allowing creativity to take the lead and guide you toward a more serene mindset.

Artistic expression is a fantastic way to practice mindfulness. Set aside some time for painting, drawing, or crafting. Gather materials you already have at home, such as paper, colors, and recycled items. Let your child lead the way, encouraging them to express their feelings and thoughts through their artwork. As you create side by side, focus on the textures, colors, and sensations of the materials in your hands. This shared experience not only nurtures creativity but also allows both of you to immerse yourselves fully in the present moment, letting go of distractions and worries.

Another wonderful activity is nature exploration. Take a leisurely walk in a park or your backyard, and encourage your child to observe the world around them. Collect leaves, stones, or flowers, and discuss their unique characteristics. As you explore, engage in conversations about the colors, shapes, and sounds of nature. This activity invites mindfulness as you both tune into the beauty of your surroundings. Simply breathing in the fresh air and soaking up the sights and sounds can significantly enhance your sense of calm and connection.

Mindful storytelling is another creative avenue to explore. Gather together and create a story that incorporates elements from your day or your child's imagination. You can take turns adding to the narrative, allowing spontaneity and creativity to flow. As you weave your tale, focus on the words, emotions, and images that arise. This practice not only sparks creativity but also cultivates a deeper awareness of your thoughts and feelings, fostering empathy and understanding between you and your child.

Finally, consider incorporating music into your mindfulness practice. Whether it's singing, dancing, or playing instruments, music can elevate your spirits and create a joyful atmosphere. Allow yourselves to be spontaneous and expressive, focusing on the rhythm and melodies. You can even explore creating your own songs together, using simple instruments or household items as percussion. This shared musical experience fosters connection and encourages both of you to be fully present, celebrating the joy of creativity in a calming way.

Chapter 7: Navigating Challenging Emotions

Recognizing Your Emotions

Recognizing your emotions is the first crucial step in cultivating mindfulness as a parent. Emotions can often feel overwhelming, especially in the whirlwind of daily life with children. However, acknowledging what you're feeling is not a sign of weakness; it's a powerful act of self-awareness. When you take a moment to pause and check in with yourself, you create space for understanding the roots of your feelings. This awareness allows you to respond to your children from a place of calm instead of reacting impulsively.

Start by identifying your emotions throughout the day. Perhaps you feel frustration when the kids refuse to cooperate during mealtime or joy when you share a laugh together. Journaling can be a helpful tool for this practice. Set aside just a few minutes each day to reflect on your feelings. Write down what you experienced, what triggered those emotions, and how they affected your interactions with your children. This simple act can illuminate patterns in your emotional responses, helping you recognize when you might need to take a step back or practice self-care.

It's also essential to embrace the full spectrum of your emotions. As parents, we often feel pressure to appear joyful and composed. However, feelings of sadness, anger, or anxiety are just as valid and deserve recognition. Instead of pushing these emotions aside, allow yourself to feel them without judgment. Remind yourself that it's okay to have tough days. Sharing your experiences with trusted friends or family members can provide relief and foster connection, reminding you that you're not alone in this journey.

Practice mindfulness techniques to enhance your emotional recognition. Techniques such as deep breathing, meditation, or simply taking a moment to observe your surroundings can ground you in the present moment. When you cultivate this practice, you'll find it easier to identify your emotions as they arise. Over time, this awareness can transform how you react in challenging situations, allowing you to approach parenting with more patience and understanding.

Lastly, remember that recognizing your emotions is a continuous journey. There will be days when you feel in tune with yourself and others when you struggle to find clarity. That's part of being human. Celebrate the small victories when you successfully pause to acknowledge your feelings and be gentle with yourself when you slip back into old patterns. Each moment is an opportunity for growth, and by recognizing your emotions, you're paving the way for a more mindful and fulfilling parenting experience. Embrace this journey with an open heart and a willingness to learn, knowing that you are doing your best for both yourself and your children.

Teaching Kids to Manage Their Feelings

Teaching kids to manage their feelings is a vital part of their emotional development, and as parents, we play a crucial role in guiding them through this process. Children experience a whirlwind of emotions daily, from joy and excitement to frustration and sadness. By helping them understand and articulate their feelings, we empower them to navigate their emotional landscape with confidence. This journey begins with creating an open and supportive environment where children feel safe to express themselves without fear of judgment.

One effective approach to teaching emotional management is through modeling our own feelings. Children are keen observers and often mimic the behavior of adults. By openly discussing our emotions, we provide them with a framework for understanding their own feelings. For instance, when we experience frustration, we can verbalize it by saying, "I'm feeling frustrated right now because I can't find my keys. I need to take a deep breath and calm down." This not only normalizes the experience of negative emotions but also demonstrates healthy coping strategies.

Incorporating mindfulness practices into our daily routines can significantly enhance our children's ability to manage their emotions. Simple techniques like deep breathing or mindfulness meditation can be introduced in a fun and engaging way. For example, we might practice "bubble breaths," where children imagine blowing bubbles as they exhale slowly. This playful approach makes the practice enjoyable while teaching them to pause and reflect before reacting to their feelings. Consistent practice helps kids develop emotional awareness, which is crucial for managing their responses to various situations.

Encouraging children to identify and label their emotions is another powerful tool. Using an emotion chart can be a fun visual aid that helps kids recognize and articulate how they feel. When they can name their emotions, they are better equipped to process and express them effectively. For instance, if a child feels angry, we can guide them to recognize that anger is a valid emotion and discuss what might have triggered it. This dialogue not only validates their feelings but also opens the door for problem-solving and finding constructive ways to cope.

In the end, fostering a sense of resilience is key in helping children manage their feelings. When we reinforce the idea that it's okay to feel a range of emotions and that they can learn from these experiences, we build their confidence in facing challenges. Encouraging them to reflect on past situations where they successfully navigated their feelings can serve as a powerful reminder of their capabilities. By nurturing resilience, we equip our children with essential life skills that will serve them well beyond childhood, helping them become emotionally intelligent and adaptable individuals.

Strategies for Staying Calm During Tantrums

Understanding how to stay calm during a child's tantrum is a vital skill that can transform a chaotic moment into an opportunity for connection and growth. When faced with a child's outburst, it's essential to remember that your calm presence can significantly influence the situation. Developing strategies to maintain your composure not only helps de-escalate the moment but also models emotional regulation for your child.

One effective strategy is to practice deep breathing. Taking a few slow, deep breaths can ground you and create a sense of serenity amidst the storm. As you inhale deeply, imagine filling your body with peace, and as you exhale, release any tension or frustration. This simple act can shift your focus away from the chaos and help you respond thoughtfully instead of reactively. Encourage yourself to pause and breathe, creating a space where you can approach your child with empathy rather than distress.

Another helpful approach is to remind yourself of the bigger picture. Children often express their overwhelming emotions through tantrums because they lack the verbal skills to articulate their feelings. By reframing the situation as a learning opportunity, you can cultivate greater patience. Focus on the idea that this moment is not just a challenge, but a chance to teach your child about emotional expression and coping mechanisms. This shift in mindset can empower you to remain calm and supportive, reinforcing your child's ability to navigate their feelings.

Establishing a mantra or affirmation can also be an effective tool during difficult moments. Phrases like "This too shall pass" or "I am here for you" can serve as gentle reminders to yourself, anchoring you in the present. When emotions run high, reciting your mantra can help quiet your mind and keep you focused on your intention to remain calm and present. This practice not only soothes you but also communicates to your child that they are safe and loved, even in their most intense moments.

Lastly, remember the power of self-care in maintaining your calm. When you prioritize your well-being, you are better equipped to handle stressful situations. Make time for activities that rejuvenate you, whether it's a quiet cup of tea, a short walk, or a few minutes of meditation. By nurturing yourself, you can cultivate a reservoir of calm that you can draw upon when your child's emotions surge. Embracing self-care as a vital part of your routine empowers you to be the mindful, patient parent you aspire to be, transforming tantrums into opportunities for connection and understanding.

Chapter 8: Mindful Transitions

Creating Routines for Smooth Transitions

Creating routines for smooth transitions is an essential practice for busy parents striving to cultivate a sense of calm in their daily lives. These routines serve as anchors, guiding both parents and children through various parts of the day with predictability and ease. Establishing a rhythm helps to alleviate the stress that often accompanies chaotic moments, allowing families to navigate changes with greater confidence and clarity.

To begin crafting effective routines, it's important to assess the specific transitions that occur in your household. Whether it's the morning rush, after-school wind-down, or bedtime preparations, identifying these key moments allows you to focus your efforts where they matter most. Consider involving your children in the process, as their input can foster a sense of ownership and excitement about the routines you create together. This collaborative approach not only strengthens family bonds but also motivates children to engage more positively during transitions.

Once you've pinpointed the transitions to address, start by outlining simple, achievable steps that can be incorporated into each routine. For instance, a morning routine might include waking up at a consistent time, having a nutritious breakfast, and setting aside a few minutes for a mindfulness exercise. These steps don't need to be elaborate; even small, intentional actions can make a significant difference in how smoothly the transition unfolds. As you establish these routines, remember to be flexible and patient with yourself and your children. Adjustments may be necessary as everyone adapts to the new structure.

Consistency is key in reinforcing these routines. Regular practice helps to instill a sense of security and familiarity, making transitions less daunting over time. Celebrate small victories along the way, acknowledging when routines are followed well. This positive reinforcement encourages children to embrace the routines and can lead to a more harmonious environment. By highlighting the benefits of these transitions, such as reduced stress and increased family time, you cultivate a shared commitment to maintaining the routines you've created.

Finally, be mindful of the emotional landscape during transitions. Recognizing that changes can be challenging for children, it's crucial to approach these moments with empathy and understanding. Use gentle reminders about the routines and offer reassurance as they adapt. By fostering an atmosphere of support and connection, you empower your family to navigate transitions with grace. Ultimately, creating routines not only brings order to the chaos but also nurtures mindfulness, helping parents and children grow together in the journey of parenting.

The Power of Rituals

Rituals have a unique power to transform the ordinary into the extraordinary. They provide a sense of structure and predictability in our busy lives, creating moments that can deepen our connections with our children. As parents, especially mothers navigating the chaos of daily responsibilities, establishing rituals can serve as a beacon of calm. These practices not only ground us but also foster a nurturing environment where our children feel secure and valued.

Incorporating simple rituals into your family routine can significantly enhance your mindfulness practice. Whether it's a bedtime story shared with a comforting cup of tea or a weekly family game night, these small traditions can create lasting memories. They allow you to slow down, breathe, and truly engage with your children. Such moments become anchors in the whirlwind of parenting, reminding us and our children of the importance of togetherness and presence.

These rituals can also serve as opportunities for teaching important values. For instance, a morning gratitude circle can cultivate appreciation and positivity, encouraging your children to express their feelings and acknowledge the good in their lives. Celebrating milestones, both big and small, through special family traditions reinforces a sense of belonging and pride. As you create these practices, you are not just making memories; you are instilling lessons that will resonate with your children for years to come.

Moreover, rituals can be a powerful tool for emotional regulation. When life feels overwhelming, returning to a familiar practice can bring comfort and stability. For example, a calming breathing exercise or a moment of silence before meals can help everyone transition from the hustle of the day to a more peaceful state. These rituals can teach children how to self-soothe and manage their emotions, equipping them with skills to navigate the challenges they will face in life.

Ultimately, the power of rituals lies in their ability to foster connection, create stability, and promote mindfulness. As busy moms, embracing these practices can transform the chaos of parenting into moments of joy and calm. By intentionally weaving rituals into your family life, you nurture not only your children's emotional well-being but also your own. Remember, it's not about perfection; it's about presence, and the simple act of showing up for each other can create a profound impact.

Mindful Bedtime Practices

Creating a mindful bedtime routine can transform the end of a busy day into a peaceful transition for both you and your child. Embracing this practice allows you to step away from the chaos of daily life and cultivate a calming environment that promotes relaxation and connection. Start by setting a consistent bedtime that works for your family. This predictability helps your child feel secure and signals that it's time to wind down. You might find that as you establish this routine, both you and your child look forward to this special time together.

Incorporating mindfulness into your bedtime practices can also enhance your child's ability to relax and settle down. Consider introducing a short breathing exercise or gentle stretching to help release the tension of the day. For example, you can guide your child through a simple deep breathing technique: inhale deeply through the nose, hold for a moment, and exhale slowly through the mouth. This not only calms their mind but also teaches them tools to manage stress in the future. Mindful breathing can become a cherished ritual that both of you can enjoy together.

Storytime is another wonderful opportunity to practice mindfulness at bedtime. Choose books that resonate with both you and your child, allowing you to explore themes of kindness, empathy, and adventure. As you read, take the time to pause and discuss the illustrations or the feelings of the characters. This engages your child's imagination while also encouraging them to express their thoughts and emotions. By sharing this reflective time, you strengthen your bond and create a nurturing space for open communication.

Creating a soothing environment plays a crucial role in your mindful bedtime practices. Dim the lights, play soft music, or use essential oils to enhance the atmosphere. Consider preparing a special bedtime ritual that might include a warm bath, a cozy blanket, or a favorite stuffed animal. These small touches can make the experience more comforting and help your child feel safe as they drift off to sleep. Remember, this is not just about helping them fall asleep; it's about fostering a sense of peace and tranquility that they can carry into their dreams.

Lastly, take a moment for yourself at the end of the bedtime routine. As your child settles into sleep, use this time to reflect on the day with gratitude. You might consider journaling or simply enjoying a cup of herbal tea. This practice not only reinforces your own mindfulness but also models healthy self-care for your child. By nurturing yourself, you are better equipped to handle the challenges of parenting. Mindful bedtime practices create a serene end to the day, nurturing both your child's spirit and your own, paving the way for a more peaceful tomorrow.

Chapter 9: Connecting with Your Partner

Prioritizing Your Relationship

Prioritizing your relationship is essential for creating a loving and supportive family environment. In the hustle and bustle of daily life, it can be easy to let your partnership take a backseat. However, nurturing your relationship not only strengthens your bond but also sets a positive example for your children. When they see you and your partner working together, communicating openly, and showing affection, they learn the importance of healthy relationships and emotional resilience.

Setting aside dedicated time for each other can significantly enhance your connection. This might mean scheduling regular date nights, even if it's just a cozy evening at home after the kids are asleep. Prioritizing this time allows you to reconnect without distractions, offering an opportunity to discuss your dreams, challenges, and the joys of parenting. It's during these moments that you can remind each other of your shared goals and the love that brought you together in the first place.

Communication is another cornerstone of a strong partnership. Practicing mindful communication—where you listen actively and express your feelings honestly—can help prevent misunderstandings and foster intimacy. Share your thoughts and concerns about parenting, and remember to celebrate your successes together. Open dialogue not only strengthens your relationship but also models healthy communication skills for your children, teaching them how to express their feelings and resolve conflicts in a constructive way.

Incorporating small gestures of appreciation into your daily life can also make a big difference. A simple "thank you" for taking out the trash or a quick note left in your partner's lunch can go a long way in affirming your commitment and care. These small acts of kindness create an atmosphere of gratitude and love, reminding both you and your partner that you are a team. This sense of partnership is vital, especially during the challenging times that parenting can bring.

In the end, remember that prioritizing your relationship is an ongoing process. It requires intention and effort from both partners. Be patient with each other and embrace the ups and downs of your journey together. By consciously making your relationship a priority, you cultivate a stable foundation for your children and create a nurturing environment where love, respect, and understanding thrive. Your commitment to each other can transform not only your relationship but also the overall family dynamic, filling your home with warmth and joy.

Communicating Mindfully as a Couple

Communicating mindfully as a couple is essential for creating a harmonious environment for your family. In the hustle and bustle of daily life, it's easy to overlook the importance of how we interact with our partners. Mindful communication fosters a deeper connection, allowing both parents to feel heard and valued. When you take the time to listen actively and express yourself thoughtfully, you set a positive example for your children and create a supportive atmosphere where everyone feels safe to express their feelings.

To begin practicing mindful communication, carve out dedicated time for meaningful conversations. This doesn't have to be a lengthy commitment; even a few minutes a day can make a significant difference. Choose a quiet moment when distractions are minimal, and focus solely on each other. Use this time to share your thoughts, feelings, and experiences without interruption. By making this a regular practice, you reinforce the idea that both partners' voices are important, which helps to cultivate a strong emotional bond.

Incorporating active listening techniques can further enhance your communication. When your partner speaks, give them your full attention. This means putting away your phone, maintaining eye contact, and nodding to show understanding. Reflect back on what you've heard to ensure clarity. This not only shows your partner that you value their perspective but also encourages them to be more open with you. By practicing active listening, you create a safe space where both partners feel comfortable sharing their thoughts and emotions without fear of judgment.

Mindful communication also involves being aware of your own emotions and reactions. When tensions arise, take a moment to pause before responding. This allows you to approach the conversation with a clear mind rather than reacting impulsively. Acknowledge your feelings and express them calmly. Using "I" statements can be particularly effective, as they focus on your experience rather than placing blame. For example, saying "I feel overwhelmed when the children are loud" conveys your feelings without making your partner defensive. This approach can lead to more productive discussions and resolutions.

Lastly, remember that maintaining a mindful communication practice takes time and patience. Be kind to yourselves as you navigate this journey together. Celebrate small victories, whether it's resolving a disagreement peacefully or simply sharing a laugh after a stressful day. By prioritizing mindful communication, you not only strengthen your partnership but also model healthy relational skills for your children. As you cultivate a more peaceful, connected home, you'll find that the chaos of parenting becomes more manageable, creating a calm space for everyone to thrive.

Shared Mindfulness Practices

Shared mindfulness practices can be a powerful tool for busy moms seeking balance and calm in their parenting journey. When you engage in mindfulness as a family, you create a nurturing environment that fosters connection and understanding among all members. These practices can help you model emotional regulation and presence, allowing your children to learn valuable life skills while deepening your bond.

One effective shared practice is mindful breathing. Set aside a few minutes each day for the whole family to sit together in a comfortable space. Encourage everyone to close their eyes and take deep, intentional breaths. You can make it more engaging by using a visual aid, like a small bell or chime, to signal when to inhale and exhale. This simple act not only calms the mind but also invites children to experience the soothing effects of mindfulness, reinforcing the importance of taking a moment to pause amidst the chaos.

Another enriching practice is mindful walking. Take a family stroll in nature or around your neighborhood, encouraging everyone to be present in the moment. As you walk, invite your children to notice the sights, sounds, and smells around them. You can turn it into a game by asking them to find specific colors or listen to different bird calls. This shared experience cultivates awareness and appreciation for the world while promoting physical activity and family bonding.

Incorporating gratitude into your family routine can also serve as a shared mindfulness practice. At dinner or bedtime, take turns sharing something you are grateful for that day. This not only helps everyone reflect on positive experiences but also teaches children to shift their focus from stressors to blessings. By practicing gratitude together, you create an atmosphere of appreciation that can transform your family's outlook on life.

Lastly, consider establishing a weekly family "mindfulness night." Dedicate this time to activities that promote mindfulness, such as yoga, meditation, or creative arts. Choose a variety of activities to keep it fun and engaging, allowing each family member to take turns leading a practice. This night can become a cherished tradition, offering a space for relaxation and connection, while reinforcing the value of mindfulness in everyday life. Embrace these shared practices, and watch as they bring your family closer together, fostering a calm and joyful home environment.

Chapter 10: Building a Supportive Community

Finding Your Tribe

Finding your tribe is an essential step in the journey of mindful parenting. As parents, particularly mothers, we often find ourselves navigating the complexities of child-rearing in isolation. The demands of daily life can make it easy to feel overwhelmed and disconnected. However, surrounding yourself with like-minded individuals who share your values and experiences can provide a sense of belonging and support that is crucial for maintaining balance. Your tribe can uplift you, validate your feelings, and offer practical advice, making the chaos of parenting feel a little more manageable.

To discover your tribe, start by exploring local community groups or online forums that focus on mindful parenting. Many parents are seeking the same connections and understanding you are, so don't hesitate to reach out. Look for parenting classes, workshops, or meetup groups in your area centered on mindfulness or holistic parenting practices. Websites and social media platforms can also be treasure troves for finding communities that resonate with your journey. Remember, the connections you forge don't have to be perfect; they simply need to offer a space where you can be yourself, share your struggles, and celebrate your victories.

Once you've found potential connections, take the step to engage with them genuinely. Share your experiences and be open about your parenting challenges. Authenticity fosters deeper connections, and your willingness to be vulnerable can encourage others to do the same. Listen actively to their stories and insights; this mutual exchange can create a sense of trust and camaraderie that enriches your parenting experience. As you build these relationships, you'll find that having people to turn to during difficult moments is invaluable, helping you feel less isolated and more empowered.

Participating in group activities can further strengthen these bonds. Consider organizing or joining regular meetups, whether they be playdates for the kids, mindfulness meditation sessions, or simple coffee chats. These gatherings not only provide emotional support but also create opportunities for shared experiences and collective learning. As you engage in mindful practices together, you'll foster an environment where everyone can grow, share their insights, and inspire one another on their parenting journeys.

Ultimately, finding your tribe is about creating a network of support that resonates with your values and parenting philosophy. A community that emphasizes mindfulness can help you cultivate patience and presence in your daily life. This tribe will remind you that you are not alone in your struggles and that together, you can navigate the chaos of parenting with grace and intention. Embrace the journey of finding your tribe, and allow these connections to nourish your spirit as you strive for calm amidst the beautiful chaos of raising children.

The Role of Playdates and Group Activities

Playdates and group activities are essential components of mindful parenting, offering children opportunities to engage socially and emotionally in a structured yet playful environment. These interactions not only foster friendships but also provide a platform for children to learn valuable life skills. As parents, facilitating these experiences can help cultivate a sense of community, allowing children to thrive in their formative years. By organizing playdates or participating in group activities, you are nurturing your child's social development while also creating a support network for yourself.

The magic of playdates lies in their ability to encourage cooperative play, where children learn to share, negotiate, and resolve conflicts. Watching your little ones navigate these interactions can be a beautiful reminder of their natural curiosity and resilience. When conflicts arise, instead of stepping in immediately, allow your child the space to explore solutions on their own. This approach not only builds their problem-solving skills but also empowers them to express their feelings and opinions. Embrace these moments as opportunities for growth, both for you and your child.

Group activities, such as sports teams, art classes, or nature clubs, provide a structured environment for children to engage with peers who share similar interests. These activities can be especially beneficial for busy parents, as they allow children to develop skills in teamwork and collaboration while they take a moment to recharge. Encouraging your child to explore different activities helps them discover their passions and strengths, fostering a sense of identity and confidence. As they interact with their peers, they are also learning the importance of diversity and inclusivity, essential values for their growth.

For parents, playdates and group activities can also serve as a vital tool for self-care. While your children participate, take the opportunity to connect with other parents, share experiences, and build friendships. These connections can provide emotional support, practical advice, or simply a moment of camaraderie in the often overwhelming journey of parenting. Remember, you are not alone in this journey; engaging with other parents can remind you of the shared challenges and joys that come with raising children.

Incorporating playdates and group activities into your family's routine creates a rich tapestry of experiences that benefit both children and parents. By fostering an environment of connection and cooperation, you are not only enhancing your child's social skills but also cultivating a mindful approach to parenting. Embrace these opportunities to strengthen relationships, support your child's development, and nurture your own well-being. Through these shared adventures, you can create lasting memories that will enrich your family's life for years to come.

Seeking Professional Support When Needed

Parenting can often feel overwhelming, and it's perfectly okay to acknowledge that you may need help along the way. Seeking professional support is a sign of strength, not weakness. Many parents face challenges that can seem insurmountable, whether it's managing stress, navigating behavioral issues, or simply balancing the demands of life. Recognizing when you need assistance is a pivotal step toward creating a more peaceful and fulfilling family environment. Embracing this journey means you are committed to your well-being and that of your children.

Professional support can come in various forms, from therapists and counselors to parenting coaches and support groups. Each of these resources offers unique perspectives and tools that can help you navigate the complexities of parenting. Therapists can provide a safe space to explore your feelings and develop coping strategies. Parenting coaches can offer practical advice tailored to your family's specific needs. Connecting with others through support groups can foster a sense of community and shared experience, reminding you that you are not alone in your struggles.

When you seek professional help, you are investing in your family's future. Mindful parenting practices often emphasize self-awareness and emotional regulation, which can be challenging to achieve without guidance. Professionals can help you cultivate these skills, enabling you to respond to your children's needs with greater patience and understanding. By learning to manage your own emotions, you can create a calmer atmosphere at home, ultimately benefiting both you and your children.

It is essential to remember that seeking help is a proactive step toward growth. Many parents have found that once they began to address their challenges with professional support, they started to notice positive changes not only in their parenting but also in their personal lives. The journey may require vulnerability, but it also fosters resilience. Each session or meeting is an opportunity to reflect, learn, and practice new techniques that can transform your parenting experience.

Embracing professional support can lead to profound changes in your family dynamics. As you learn and grow, you will likely find that your relationships with your children become more connected and harmonious. By prioritizing your mental and emotional health, you are setting a powerful example for your children about the importance of self-care and seeking help when needed. Remember, the path to calm parenting is not a solitary one; it is filled with opportunities for support, growth, and connection.

Chapter 11: Cultivating Gratitude and Joy

Daily Gratitude Practices

Daily gratitude practices can transform the way you approach parenting and life in general. By intentionally focusing on what you appreciate, you cultivate a positive mindset that can help reduce stress and enhance your overall well-being. As busy moms, it can be easy to get caught up in the chaos of daily responsibilities, but taking time to acknowledge the good things in your life can provide a sense of calm amidst the storms of parenting.

One simple yet effective practice is to start or end your day with a gratitude journal. Each morning or evening, take a few moments to reflect on three things you are thankful for. They can be as simple as a warm cup of coffee, a hug from your child, or the sun shining through your window. Writing these moments down not only solidifies them in your memory but also serves as a reminder of the positivity that exists in your life. Over time, this practice can shift your focus from what's lacking to what's abundant, nurturing a mindset of appreciation.

Another engaging way to incorporate gratitude into your daily routine is through family discussions. During dinner or before bedtime, encourage each family member to share something they are grateful for. This not only fosters a sense of connection among family members but also teaches your children the importance of recognizing and valuing the good in their lives. As they witness you expressing gratitude, they are more likely to adopt this practice themselves, creating a ripple effect of positivity within your household.

Mindfulness exercises can also enhance your gratitude practice. Take a few minutes each day to sit quietly and focus on your breath, allowing yourself to become aware of your surroundings and the sensations in your body. As thoughts of stress and chaos arise, gently redirect your mind to what you appreciate about your day or your family. This mindful approach helps anchor your thoughts in the present moment, making it easier to recognize and embrace gratitude, even during challenging times.

Lastly, consider creating visual reminders of gratitude around your home. This could be a family gratitude board where you pin notes of appreciation or a jar where each family member can drop in notes of gratitude throughout the week. These tangible reminders will not only elevate your mood but also serve as a beautiful testament to the love and joy present in your life. By integrating these daily gratitude practices, you will cultivate a more peaceful and fulfilling parenting experience, transforming chaos into calm.

Celebrating Small Wins

Celebrating small wins is an essential practice in the journey of mindful parenting. In the hustle and bustle of daily life, it can be easy to overlook the little victories that occur throughout the day. These moments, whether it's a child finally tying their shoes independently, sharing a laugh during breakfast, or successfully navigating a challenging conversation, deserve to be acknowledged and celebrated. By recognizing these achievements, parents not only boost their own morale but also foster a positive environment for their children, instilling a sense of accomplishment and confidence.

When we take the time to celebrate small wins, we shift our focus from what still needs to be done to what has already been achieved. This perspective change is powerful. It allows us to cultivate gratitude and appreciation for the everyday moments that bring joy and connection. Consider setting aside a few moments each evening to reflect on the day's highlights, no matter how minor they may seem. This practice can transform your mindset and create a more positive atmosphere in your home, making it easier to navigate the challenges that arise.

Integrating celebrations into daily routines can be simple and enjoyable. You might create a small ritual, such as a family high-five after completing chores or sharing a "win of the day" at the dinner table. These rituals not only provide an opportunity to recognize achievements but also strengthen family bonds. They encourage open communication and help children understand the value of celebrating their efforts, no matter how small. This can lead to increased motivation and a willingness to tackle new challenges together.

Additionally, celebrating small wins can serve as a reminder to practice self-compassion as parents. It's easy to fall into the trap of self-criticism when things don't go as planned. By acknowledging your own small victories, whether it's managing to stay calm during a tantrum or making a nutritious meal, you reinforce the idea that you are doing your best. This self-acknowledgment is crucial for maintaining mental well-being and helps prevent feelings of burnout that can occur in the demanding role of parenting.

Ultimately, embracing and celebrating small wins creates a ripple effect, enriching the family dynamic and nurturing a positive mindset. Every day presents numerous opportunities to recognize achievements, no matter how small. By focusing on these moments, you not only enhance your own parenting experience but also teach your children the importance of resilience and appreciation. In this mindful journey, let us honor the small wins that pave the way for greater successes, turning chaos into calm, one celebration at a time.

Finding Joy in Everyday Moments

Finding joy in everyday moments is a transformative practice that can significantly enhance your experience as a parent. In the hustle and bustle of daily life, it's easy to overlook the simple pleasures that surround us. As busy moms, we often find ourselves caught up in a whirlwind of responsibilities, from school runs to meal prep, and in this chaos, we might forget to pause and appreciate the little things. By consciously choosing to embrace joy in these moments, we can cultivate a deeper connection with our children and foster a more positive family environment.

One of the simplest ways to find joy is to practice mindfulness. This means being fully present in the moment, whether you're watching your child play, sharing a meal, or reading a bedtime story. Instead of letting your thoughts drift to the next task on your to-do list, try to immerse yourself in the experience at hand. Pay attention to the sounds, sights, and feelings around you. Notice the laughter of your children, the warmth of their hugs, or even the smell of their favorite snacks. These sensory experiences can bring a profound sense of happiness and fulfillment that often goes unnoticed amidst our busy lives.

Creating rituals can also enhance your ability to find joy in everyday moments. Consider establishing small routines that you look forward to, such as family game nights or weekend nature walks. These rituals not only provide structure but also become cherished traditions that your family can bond over. They create opportunities for connection and laughter, reminding everyone that joy can be found in shared experiences. The anticipation of these moments can bring a sense of excitement and joy that permeates your days, making even the mundane feel special.

Remember, joy is not always about grand gestures or special occasions. It can be found in the smallest of actions and interactions. A spontaneous dance party in the kitchen, a cozy cuddle session on the couch, or even just sharing a smile with your child can light up your day. These fleeting moments often hold the most significance, and by acknowledging them, you create a positive atmosphere that encourages love and appreciation. Encourage your children to recognize and celebrate these moments too, fostering a family culture where joy is always valued.

In the end, it's essential to be compassionate with yourself. Parenting is a journey filled with ups and downs, and it's perfectly normal to feel overwhelmed at times. Embrace the idea that finding joy is a practice, not a destination. Allow yourself to feel the full range of emotions that come with parenting, and remember that it's okay to seek joy amidst challenges. By nurturing an attitude of gratitude and mindfulness, you will find yourself more equipped to experience the joy that each day has to offer, ultimately transforming your parenting experience into one filled with love and connection.

Chapter 12: Sustaining Mindfulness in Busy Lives

Overcoming Obstacles to Mindfulness

Overcoming obstacles to mindfulness is an essential journey for parents striving to cultivate a sense of calm in their chaotic lives. Many mothers face numerous distractions, both external and internal, that can make it challenging to practice mindfulness consistently. Recognizing these obstacles is the first step toward overcoming them. By acknowledging that distractions are a natural part of parenting, you can begin to shift your perspective and approach mindfulness with a more forgiving attitude. Embracing the notion that it's okay to face challenges can empower you to find solutions tailored to your unique circumstances.

One common challenge is the overwhelming nature of daily responsibilities. From juggling work commitments to managing household tasks, it can feel impossible to carve out time for mindfulness. However, it's important to remember that mindfulness doesn't have to be a lengthy practice. Even a few moments of intentional breathing or a short meditation can make a significant difference in your day. Consider incorporating these practices into existing routines, like taking a mindful moment while preparing meals or during a break at work. These small adjustments can gradually transform your mindset and help you cultivate mindfulness amidst the chaos.

Another obstacle many parents encounter is the struggle with self-judgment. It's easy to feel guilty or inadequate when trying to practice mindfulness, especially when distractions arise or when you find it hard to concentrate. It's crucial to approach mindfulness with compassion for yourself. Understand that mindfulness is not about achieving perfection but about being present in the moment. Celebrate your efforts, no matter how small, and remind yourself that every attempt is a step forward. By reframing your mindset, you can create a more supportive environment for your mindfulness journey.

Environmental factors can also pose significant challenges to mindfulness. A noisy household, constant interruptions, or a busy schedule can derail your efforts to find peace. To address this, consider creating a designated mindfulness space in your home, however small, where you can retreat for a few moments of quiet. This space can be as simple as a cozy corner with a cushion or a chair where you can practice breathing exercises or meditation. Having a physical space dedicated to mindfulness can serve as a reminder to prioritize your mental well-being, making it easier to escape the chaos for a few moments each day.

Finally, involving your children in mindfulness practices can be a powerful way to overcome obstacles while fostering a sense of calm for the entire family. Engaging in activities like mindful breathing, simple yoga poses, or even nature walks together can not only introduce mindfulness to their lives but also create cherished family moments. By making mindfulness a shared experience, you not only enrich your parenting journey but also model the importance of self-care to your children. Remember, the path to mindfulness is not a destination but a continuous journey, and with each small step, you can transform chaos into calm, both for yourself and your family.

Incorporating Mindfulness into Daily Tasks

Incorporating mindfulness into daily tasks can transform the way parents approach their responsibilities, creating a more serene environment for both themselves and their children. Mindfulness is about being present in the moment, and it can be seamlessly integrated into the routine activities of parenting. Whether you are preparing meals, helping with homework, or simply enjoying a quiet moment, each task offers an opportunity to practice mindfulness. This not only enhances your connection to the present but also sets a powerful example for your children, teaching them the value of being aware and engaged in their lives.

One of the simplest ways to start incorporating mindfulness is by focusing on your breath. Before beginning any daily task, take a moment to inhale deeply, fill your lungs with air, and then exhale slowly. This brief pause can help ground you, clearing your mind of distractions. For instance, while washing dishes, concentrate on the sensation of water on your hands, the sound of the dishes clinking, and the warmth of the soap. By fully immersing yourself in the task at hand, you not only make the activity more enjoyable but also cultivate a sense of calm that can ripple through your entire day.

Another effective practice is to turn routine chores into mindful moments. While folding laundry, instead of rushing through the task, take time to appreciate the textures and colors of the clothes. Think about the memories associated with each item, whether it's a favorite shirt or a cozy blanket. This shift from a mundane chore to a reflective activity can help foster gratitude and joy in everyday life. Engaging with tasks on this deeper level allows you to find beauty in the ordinary and encourages your children to appreciate their surroundings as well.

Mindfulness can also be integrated into interactions with your children during daily routines. When helping with homework or reading a bedtime story, practice active listening. Put aside distractions, make eye contact, and truly engage with what your child is saying. This not only strengthens your bond but also teaches your child the importance of mindfulness in communication. By modeling this behavior, you encourage them to be present in their own interactions, fostering empathy and understanding in their relationships.

Lastly, remember that incorporating mindfulness is a journey, not a destination. It's normal to have moments of distraction or chaos—embrace them without judgment. Celebrate small successes and acknowledge how even brief moments of mindfulness can create a more peaceful atmosphere in your home. By weaving mindfulness into your daily tasks, you cultivate a nurturing environment that supports both your well-being and that of your children, ultimately guiding your family from chaos to calm.

Creating a Lifelong Mindfulness Practice

Creating a lifelong mindfulness practice is a rewarding journey for parents, especially for busy moms who often juggle multiple responsibilities. Establishing this practice can transform the way you approach parenting and life in general. It begins with small, intentional actions that can be integrated into your daily routine. Start by carving out just a few minutes each day for mindfulness. This can be as simple as focusing on your breath while you sip your morning coffee or taking a moment to appreciate the world around you as you walk with your child. These small moments create a foundation for a more mindful existence.

As you grow more comfortable with these brief moments of mindfulness, consider incorporating them into your family activities. Engage your children in mindful practices, such as focusing on the sensations of eating a meal together or noticing the sounds of nature during a family walk. By modeling mindfulness, you not only enhance your own practice but also instill valuable skills in your children. This shared experience fosters a deeper connection within your family and helps everyone develop greater awareness and presence, enriching your family life.

To solidify your mindfulness practice, explore various techniques and find what resonates with you and your family. Guided meditations, mindful breathing exercises, or yoga sessions can offer different ways to cultivate mindfulness. Encourage your children to participate in activities that promote mindfulness, such as coloring or playing with sensory materials. These practices can serve as enjoyable ways to relax and reset, allowing you to embrace the present moment and cultivate a sense of calm amidst the chaos of parenting.

Consistency is key in creating a lifelong mindfulness practice. Try to set aside dedicated time each week for mindfulness activities, whether individually or as a family. This could be a Sunday evening ritual of meditation or mindfulness games that everyone looks forward to. As you establish this routine, it becomes a cherished part of your family life, providing a sense of stability and peace that can be particularly nurturing in the hectic pace of modern parenting.

Remember, mindfulness is a journey, not a destination. There will be days when it feels challenging to maintain your practice, and that's perfectly okay. Embrace those moments with self-compassion and understanding. Celebrate your progress, no matter how small, and remind yourself that every effort counts. By committing to a lifelong mindfulness practice, you are not only nurturing your own well-being but also creating a legacy of awareness and calm that will benefit your children for years to come.

Chapter 13: Conclusion

In conclusion, this book has explored the fundamental themes of resilience, personal growth, and the power of community. We have examined the challenges faced by the characters, the lessons learned through their journeys, and the impact of their relationships on their development. Each chapter has served to illustrate the importance of perseverance and the strength found in vulnerability.

As you reflect on these insights, remember that every challenge you encounter is an opportunity for growth. Embrace your journey, lean on your community, and know that you have the strength to overcome obstacles. Keep moving forward with courage and determination.

If you found value in this book or enjoyed it, I would greatly appreciate it if you could take a moment to leave a review. Your feedback not only helps me improve, but also assists other readers in finding this work. Thank you for being part of this journey.

www.ingramcontent.com/pod-product-compliance
Lightning Source LLC
Chambersburg PA
CBHW051818250726
48659CB00005B/1543